Calories Counter

How To Get Skinny Using The Latest Technology

Written by
K. L. Becker

Disclaimer

This publication is designed to provide accurate and authoritative information in regard to the subject matter covered. It is sold with the understanding that the publisher is not engaged in rendering health, legal, nutritional, accounting, or other professional services. If professional advice or other expert assistance is required, the services of a competent professional person should be sought. Designated trademarks and brands are the property of their respective owners.

Table of Contents

Introduction

If you are thinking about losing weight by counting calories or have tried and could not make it work I think I have some tips, tricks and resources that will be helpful in your struggle to lose weight. Many people have tried to count calories and have become frustrated with the complexity, difficulty in getting it right and the time and effort it takes to make calorie counting work effectively. Well the good news is there is new and ever improving technology that makes this daunting task much easier than when your grandmother tried counting calories with a scale, information on labels, a calculator and notebook.

After some initial observations about the increasing problem of obesity and why many of us are having difficulty with diets and dieting, I will give you a few suggestions about how to approach losing weight with calorie counting and how to improve the overall process of losing weight by counting calories.

This book goes on to give you ideas of where you can go to start or improve calorie counting in your weight loss program. If you are in tune with using the web there are a couple of suggested websites where you will find comprehensive online calorie counting programs allowing you to log and track not only the calories you eat but also the calories you burn. Also included is a review of a popular app you can use on your Smartphone.

There also is some useful information about what is available on "wrist watch" type devices for sophisticated counting and tracking of calories burned during workouts and normal daily activities such as shopping and housework.

Lastly, I wrap it up with what you REALLY need to do to be successful with counting calories with the goal of losing weight.

This is not a listing of foods and calorie counts but where to find and how to effectively use some great resources out there that have HUGE calorie databases with sophisticated tracking technology and, for the most part, they are FREE!

Don't forget to download your free report!

http://www.weightlossextrabonus.com

Chapter 1

Sadly, We Are Becoming Obese

Losing weight has been frustrating for a vast majority of individuals. No matter what kind of exercise they do, or no matter what diet plan they follow, a lot of people still fail to reach their goals.

In fact, the problem is becoming much bigger than just not achieving weight loss goals. There is an obesity epidemic in our society that's getting worse every year. More and more of us have an obese body mass index (BMI) of 30 plus. The latest statistics show that there are 58 million overweight Americans with 40 million classified as obese and 3 million morbidly obese. Even a large number of our children are grossly obese. Why is this happening?

Is It What We Are Eating?

Some researchers conclude that along with the lack of exercise, the problem is with the food we eat. Processed food, they say, is full of added sugar, salt and fat to make it taste better. If fact, some research concludes that 70% of the calories we consume are from processed foods and that currently the average American spends less than thirty minutes per day in the kitchen actually cooking the food they eat. We are spending more time watching cooking shows than we are actually cooking meals we eat. This means that we are consuming mostly processed food calories that are not very nutritious in addition to being way too fattening.

Is It All Very Confusing And Just Too Hard?

If you are trying to lose weight you may be asking questions like "Why can't I lose weight no matter how hard I try? What food should I eat and what shouldn't I eat in order to achieve my weight loss goal? How much should I eat and when? What about nutrients? Are they important?"

Trying to get the best diet for you as a unique individual can be a daunting and confusing journey. If you are truly trying to achieve a diet that is going to be sustainable over your lifetime, it should not subject you to "Yo-Yo" crash or starvation diets that might allow you to lose weight in the short run. But when you eventually can't continue to starve yourself any longer, the weight just "balloons" back on and you end up in worse shape than if you had not started on the crazy diet to begin with.

Or, maybe you have a great diet but you can't stop the cheating.

Are You A Diet Cheater?
While some of us can have a "medical addiction" to food that can be just as debilitating as a drug or alcohol addiction, most of us are just "diet cheaters" without the self-discipline to do what it takes to lose weight. We are what I call "diet cheaters"

Chapter 2

What Do I Mean By Diet Cheating?

I mean eating that candy bar or drinking that sugary soft drink definitely not on our weight loss plan full well knowing you have just broken the rules so critical to follow if you are going to have any chance to lose the weight you so desperately want to lose.

When we can hide our diet cheating and no one will know except us, then cheating is too easy and there is no pain or punishment for doing so.

Why Many High Priced Diet Programs FAIL!

This is precisely why diet programs where you "weigh in" every week with other dieters have been so successful. There is at least the pain of embarrassment or the thought that the very expensive price tag for buying into the diet program is just getting wasted.

However, for many this isn't enough punishment and the dropout rate from most of these very expensive diet programs remains very high

Chapter 3

No Pain? Then You Will Gain

You ask: "Why do I need punishment in my diet?" It's not that we need punishment in the strict sense of the word. Simply we need our brain to be conditioned to "feel" the consequence (or the pain if you like) of cheating on our diet and we need to feel it now rather than later.

When weight gain happens gradually there is an emotional disconnect between consuming more calories than you burn off every day and the eventual "pain" of being overweight. One day we wake up "fat" and wonder "How in the world did THIS happen? I haven't been eating more than normal. Have I? "

One More Little Cookie Won't Hurt
In other words, the pain of being overweight is far removed or delayed from the behavior of overeating. Your mind reasons: "One more little cookie is not going to hurt".

This is not the case when you accidentally put your hand directly on the hot burner of your cooking stove in the kitchen. Here the pain is right now and you are logically and more importantly "emotionally" conditioned to not do this again. It hurts and it hurts right now!

With dieting how can we get the same "painful" effect when we cheat ourselves out of the rewards of losing weight and looking great because cheating is too easy and has no such immediate physical pain to stop us from doing it?

Now I'm not suggesting that you put your hand on a hot stove every time you fall off of your diet. However, your mind needs to know that when you do "cheat" there is going to be an unpleasant consequence. More on this later...stay tuned we are going to cover this in detail.

Chapter 4

Condition Your Cheating Mind

How do we condition our mind so that there is immediate punishment rather than reward for cheating on our diet?

Well a good start is to use something visual like a scorecard so when your scorecard is constantly in "failing or success" status and you look at it every time you put something in your mouth, your mind will eventually get conditioned to make the connection between what you eat now and what your weight will be eventually.

If your score says you are eating too much and your weight is gaining then unless you are in a state of "complete denial" there is NO DENYING you are not following your diet plan.

The next psychological step is to actually be concerned enough about it to get back on track.

Your Diet Scorecard

An immediate visual reward or punishment mechanism that will condition your mind to follow your diet plan is what you need.

What would this look like? A visual display will work as long as it is very easy to see, to use and to understand exactly what is going on with your caloric intake vs. burn rate daily along with each meal and snack you choose to eat.

Chapter 5

Counting Calories With Technology

This "diet scorecard" should have the capability to show trend lines that exactly measure when your calorie intake is less than what you are burning with exercise and other daily activities.

It must show you that you are successfully losing weight and how much. Or, that you are failing and how badly with each meal and drink that you decide to ingest.

Charts with trend lines are great visual tools. This calorie/exercise counter/calculator should also be able to calculate and display changes in your body mass index (BMI).

Asking How Hungry You Are At Meal Time

Another feature this diet management tool might have is hunger level meal planning. If you have a tool that can help you plan meals depending on how hungry you are, you will be able to lose weight without the hunger pain and rollercoaster emotions of crash or fad diets. You should not eat a big meal if you are not hungry since this will add unnecessary calories. On the other hand eating too little of the right foods at meal time when you are hungrier than normal will put you at risk of snacking on the wrong foods in between meals.

Wouldn't it be nice if weight loss were pleasurable and losing weight daily along with looking more attractive actually became easy? What a concept!

What kinds of calories counters are available and what is best for your diet plan, life style and technological capability? Let's take a look.

Chapter 6

Simple Calories Counters

There are a number of online websites, software applications, Smartphone apps and hand held electronic devices that offer calories counting. Many free online versions will only add what food items you enter and display the total calorie count.

Useful and Simple To Use Websites but...
Some websites will calculate then compare the calories contained in two different food items. For example, you can enter potatoes chips vs. Cheetos then compare the calorie count for each. This is kind of fun to do. Go to twofoods.com and give it try.

There are different methods to count calories and the most common are online calorie calculators. You can find a lot of these calculators out there and they're pretty simple to use. What you do to use them is to put in the meals you've eaten, including liquids, and they will give you the approximate amount of calories that you've had for the entire day.

Some online calculators also allow you to see the total amount of calories you've had for the day, and how many calories are left for the entire week. This is an effective method of watching the food that you eat and definitely one of the best ways to lose those excess pounds if you are religious about inputting ALL of the data. However, are you online every time you put something in your mouth?

Your Score Is Important… Get What You Need
What you really need is a sophisticated system that cannot only calculate calorie intake and burn data but will also store the data and display it in such a way as to show you whether you are gaining or burning calories every day and over an extended period of time at your fingertips…no matter where you are or what time of the day or night it is. Before we get into this however, let's start by looking at what you should track no matter how you keep track of it.

Chapter 7

Let's Start With The Basics

Whether you use a handwritten calorie counter and exercise diary to keep score or a high tech Smartphone app, what should you keep track of at the minimum?

The best rule of thumb when you're trying to lose weight is to always remember that you can't intake more calories than you can burn. Calories are necessary - they provide you with the energy that you need to get through the day, but excess or unburned calories will eventually turn into fat deposits, causing weight gain.

Calories Eaten – Calories Burned

So as you add in the calories you eat and subtract out the calories you burn, if you look at your daily score card and it says 3500 calories in and 2000 calories burned, you are not burning off calories you are gaining weight!

On the other hand, during that same day if you burn off let's say 4000 calories that day you will be losing weight at the rate of about one pound every 7 days.

Just remember that it takes around 2000 calories ingested each day for a typical active adult to maintain their current body weight. This is just a "rule of thumb" and is highly dependent on your current weight, age, gender, health, activity level and a number of other factors.

You are going to have to determine how many calories you need to burn off over what you have eaten every day to reach your weight loss goal. We will get into this basic concept later but just know that there are two ways to achieve a daily deficit necessary for your body to lose weight.

You can either cut back on the amount of calories you eat or increase the number of calories you burn off every day. If you are serious about weight loss, you will do both and keep an accurate record regarding both. How can you know if you are progressing if you don't "keep score"? It is really that simple.

Your Plan Must Fit Your Individual Situation
Your optimal calorie deficiency that will be the correct number for you to achieve your weight loss goal is highly dependent on your individual circumstance. You will need to take your individual age, gender, height, current weight and fitness level into account when determining how much total weight you want to lose and how fast you want to lose it. Your Current health status is very important. Don't try to lose too much weight too quickly and jeopardize your health. Also, if you are pregnant, remember you are eating for two people!

A good place to start is a consultation with your personal doctor. Your doctor should be able to advise you about what your safe personal weight loss goals should be given the state of your health. There are good online resources available to you in determining the calories your body needs to maintain its current weight and how much you will need to "exercise off" every day in order to lose weight. We will get into these resources in more detail later in this book.

When Your Weight Loss Plan Is Finalized
You really need to figure out how many calories are in the foods you eat every day. If you are doing this with paper and pen, you will have to find good reference sources showing how many calories are in the food you eat every day. If you are not continuously online then you will have to carry a thick reference manual with calorie data per portion size wherever you go or make use of "always with you" high tech tools we will review later.

If You Have To Write It Down In a Diet Diary
There are different products being introduced in the market everyday however the traditional handwritten way can still work for anyone. The traditional log book or diet journal method still allows anyone to watch what they eat and learn how to count calories being careful to not take in more than what they can burn each day, each week, each month. But doing it this way is similar to using a typewriter vs. a word processor.

If you choose to write it all down then get a notebook that is small enough to carry around yet with enough pages so that you can devote one page per day. Then you will have to make sure that you log in everything that goes into your mouth not only meals but also snacks, beverages, sauces, butter, etc., even everything that is used to prepare and spice up your meals.

You may have the choice to calculate and record the calorie count of the meals and snacks you are eating at the time you consume them by looking at the label on the package or tin can that discloses calorie and nutrition data.

If You Are Reading Labels
Recording calorie count and nutritional information from labels on tin cans and packages can be somewhat tricky if you are not aware of what exactly to look for.

The first task of getting this right is to make sure you locate and thoroughly understand the serving size. So if your food item package says two servings and the calorie information on the label is for the entire package, if you eat only one serving then all calorie count information, etc. on the label needs to be cut in half. This, however, is not usually the problem.

The problem is almost always in the other direction. You eat four rather than two servings and the label calorie count on the package is per serving. This can get harder to measure when the serving size is not in real obvious units such as pieces but rather is labeled something like "scoops". I'm sure my scoop is much smaller than YOUR scoop...right?

Many times you will find that it is possible to measure a serving size by weighing it or by using a measuring cup. In other words, the label will have the portion size in grams or ounces, even cups. Of course this means you will have to have an accurate scale to weigh your food and it is not really practical to weigh food when you are at a restaurant or invited out to eat at your friends or family's house.

Another thing to watch out for on the label is "servings per container". This may not be a real precise measurement. If you are not careful about measuring out your serving when you eat it, you can be way off with the calorie count. Try to see how many cups or grams or pieces are in one container and divide by what you think you would eat for a normal serving. You are attempting to log in an accurate calorie count per serving. Sometimes the manufacturer will provide you with several measurements per container.

If you are unable to find the information you are looking for on labels, you may want to purchase a calorie reference book allowing you to look up the calorie information you need.

The Complete Book of Food Counts
A good one to check out is The Complete Book of Food Counts, published by Random House, Author Corrine T. Netzer. This is a complete reference manual that is recommended by many doctors and dieticians alike for their patients desperately trying to stay on a diet.

The book has a long history going back to 1988 and has had several updates since the original publication and has been released eight times since then. This huge calorie and nutrition manual contains not only calorie data but other information on carbs, fat, cholesterol content, salt level, protein and fiber measured either in milligrams or grams for every dish or food items listed whether consumed in fast food restaurants or cooked from scratch at home.

Finding Your Calorie Count Online
Many online sites have a large database of calorie data at your finger tips such as

www.acaloriecounter.com

Going through the routine at each meal and keeping a running count during the day may help you develop the discipline you will need to adequately do the work necessary for accurate calories counting. Otherwise, you are going to have to make sure that you go through the routine of finding the calorie count of the foods you ingested during the day and doing the calculating and recording once during the evening.

You will also have to do the same for the calories you burn by recording the exercise and normal daily activities such as housework or grocery shopping that burn calories.

How Can You Make This As Easy As Possible?

It's this simple, people with less activity need fewer calories, and people who do more physical activities need more calories. It's a matter of what is the simplest and easiest way to keep track of net daily calories that works best for you and your level of technical resourcefulness.

Now the question is, how do you count the calories that you eat and burn and get to the answers fast and easily so that calculating and logging calories eaten and calories burned is not a time consuming, difficult hassle requiring several steps, reading labels, carrying reference and note books or logging onto the Internet with every bite of food or step you take? This much effort could eventually lead to giving up because it's just too hard to do and it is way too easy just to give it up.

Chapter 8

Online Calories Counting

You can find good diet calculators and counters online. I obviously can't review or suggest all or even several of the great websites that are currently online to help you with your calories counting requirements. If you are online you probably know how to conduct a search that will result in several websites for you to test out. However, you can start by testing this one out.

The Food-o-Meter
A good one to start with is WebMD's Food-o-Meter. This gives you a great selection of items that are clickable in a drop down menu and you can input portion sizes and number of servings to get as accurate as possible.

The Fit-o-Meter

What I like about this resource is that you have available both sides of the equation with WebMD's Fit-o-Meter. Again just choose the exercise you are going to do, for an example, walking up stairs. You will then be taken to twelve choices about how you are going to do it…with moderate loads of say 15 lbs, moving household items up the stairs or just carrying groceries? Input your weight and duration of time doing the exercise, then click the calculate button to find out how many calories this exercise will burn. Add it to your overall activity summary and you have a way to keep track of your calories burned for the day.

The Food & Fitness Planner

You can even use this site as your overall calories counting system by starting with the Food & Fitness Planner. By inputting your basic personal data such as gender, weight, birth date and height you will start with what should be your overall weight and body mass index presented in ranges.

The tool will then help you plan your weight loss goal and calculate a recommendation of how best to achieve that goal. Lastly, you can log your food and exercise activities and keep track of your progress showing you how your weight has changed over the time you have used the system. If the foods or specific exercises are not already available for you conveniently by choosing them, then by using drop down menus you can input your own custom items both in the food and exercise categories.

This system also can keep track of nutrients such as fat, cholesterol, salt, carbohydrates, sugar and others.

Another great online resource to help you design a weight loss program and keep track of your daily calories count can be found at:

www.livestrong.com/thedailyplate

Exercise can also be tracked.

So here you go with two great online places to get started or at least check out if you decide that your PC is going to be the tool of choice for calories counting and tracking. Next is the best available technology to use in my opinion.

Chapter 9

Using The Best Technology

Although online calories counters and calculators or handwritten diet diaries and food calorie manuals are okay, there are many individuals who prefer using their Smartphone for as many tasks as they can, since they barely stay at home yet still want the convenience and ease of utilizing the best and latest mobile technology.

Nowadays, you can find mobile applications that allow you to key in your realistic weight loss goal - put in your current weight, how much you want to lose within a week, and the application will tell you how many calories you should eat and burn to achieve your goal. However, some apps available offer even much more than this.

The Calorie Counter Smartphone App

As an example, there is a highly rated app that runs on the Android and iPhone platforms (among others) by MyFitnessPal.com called Calorie Counter offering many useful features. It has fully functional features that include food and exercise diaries, a diet calendar and a weight tracker.

Logging Your Calories Count with This App

In the food diary function you can log your daily food calorie intake several ways. First, there is a drop down menu of foods you find when doing a search and you can add them to your breakfast, lunch, dinner or snack meals by clicking a plus button. Or, choose foods by looking in categories including restaurants or even grocery brand names.

One of the greatest features of this app is your ability to scan bar codes. How cool is that! Who needs to agonize over searching? Just scan the bar code right on the package and enter your portion size! You can also save frequently eaten foods or whole meals as we tend to eat the same things again and again.

Your Exercise Diary

This feature will allow you to estimate the number of calories you have burned throughout the day including sleeping or resting. The list of exercise activities is very extensive allowing you to be as accurate as possible in helping to determine the calories you eat and burn per day with each meal you eat and exercise you do.

Your Diet Calendar and Weight Tracker

These valuable features are where your calories counting work allows you to "keep score" and feel good about whether you are winning or losing: being rewarded or punished in the war of weight loss you are waging.

Watch your net calorie count each day. Are you burning more than you are eating? Your weight tracker will allow you to see which exercise activities and foods are working for you and which ones are working against you.

If you want, you can synchronize your app data with an online account that provides even more features and information.

The Best Part

There are some additional features that are cool like finding where to buy a food item you want at the nearest grocery with Google maps (android version) and what other food products are offered by the brand that you frequently eat.

However, the Best Part: This App is **FREE** as in No Cost to Download and use! As Always, be sure to read and thoroughly understand the privacy statement!

The android version is available on Google Play and the iPhone version can be downloaded from iTunes. You can find links to download this app at:

www.weightlossextrabonus.com/resources

Chapter 10

Calorie Burn Counter On Your Wrist

If you don't own a Smartphone and still want the convenience of anywhere, anytime, then one alternative you have is to buy a calories counter wrist watch. These can be effective for the exercise part of your calories counting system and relatively inexpensive. Many are really just sophisticated pedometers. Most will have a stopwatch and can display the time and date like a traditional wrist watch.

Pricey Models

They also can be highly sophisticated, feature rich and pretty darned expensive. Mostly what you will find will be models that are oriented toward burning calories rather than inputting meals and snacks as some models have a heart rate monitor and can indicate calories you are burning according to how fast your heart is beating. Some models include a chest strap and heart monitor that is attached to your chest.

These counters are good when you are running as many of them will keep track of pace, distance and time parameters.

Some of the higher end models include GPS functionality and an AM/FM radio. Some models allow you to upload data to a computer software program that can calculate parameters for the purposes of displaying charts and graphs of your calorie burning activities.

The Real Advantages Of Using One

One of the advantages of using a calorie counter wrist watch is that it will provide motivation to reach goals during your exercise periods that you may characterize as "workouts". The rate at which you are burning calories may not be enough for you to achieve your net calorie loss for the day and this will be obvious if you are wearing a watch showing what you are actually burning during your workout. You may need to create a more intense workout routine, spend more time doing your current exercise of choice or do it more often during the day.

If you do adjust your activity based on the feedback you are getting from your wrist counter, it is extremely rewarding to visually see with your own two eyes the achievement of your calorie burn goal both for your workout sessions and for the entire day.

Only Half Of What You Need To Keep Track Of

Even though all of the features of the watch type calories counter can be very useful in precisely keeping track of your exercise and calories burned per day, most models really only deal with half of the equation. You still need to calculate and log what your caloric intake is daily. You will not lose weight even if you are exercising all day long but still eating more calories than you burn!

A Closer Look At A Specific Device

One wrist band system to check out is the UP band made by Jawbone. The great part about this system is that, depending upon your Smartphone's operating system, all of the data you collect with it can be integrated with the data captured by your Calorie Counter App. The band is small, lightweight and comfortable to wear. It is also water resistant and does not need to be taken off when you are taking a shower.

Tracking Exercises with The UP

Features that some find useful are activity logging that is "step based". This function will keep track not only of calories burned but also distance, if running or walking, time spent and intensity. You can also choose other activities that aren't necessarily step based but are more machine or standing based, as an example, the category cardio, allows you to enter a higher calorie burn rate than what is preprogrammed into the band.

Even While You Sleep

You can keep track of sleep that not only includes "deep" periods but light sleep as well and there is a separate "power" nap feature that will awake you in a little over 25 minutes, the optimal time for a power nap.

Too Much Couch Time?

A timer can be set to vibrate if you have prolonged "couch potato" periods through the day. You can even keep track of your "moods" throughout the day to discover what triggers good and bad moods throughout your day and night..."here comes the boss" or "FAC is getting close!"

Track Food Also

Here is a great feature not normally found on wrist type devices. If you don't want to have to hassle with two apps or an app, a website and a wrist device you can also use this device to count the calories you eat. It may not have the sophistication of some other calorie counter apps or website programs but, if you want, you can use it to track both sides...calories in and calories burned making this particular wrist device more than only half of what you need.

Uploading Your Data

In order to upload data you plug the UP wrist band into the microphone outlet on your Smartphone. You can buy this device from several vendors including eBay and Amazon in addition to buying it directly from Jawbone.

The Jawbone UP is only one of many wrist calorie counter devices on the market. I suggest you do your own research and read several consumer reviews to find the perfect device for your individual need.

Chapter 11

More Than Counting Calories

Don't fall into the trap of thinking that as long as you are counting calories that you can eat whatever you want. In other words your cheating mind might think "Well, I have a large calorie deficiency today because I have skipped breakfast and lunch and ate a very small dinner and included an extra workout period therefore now I can pig out on ice cream for dessert and still make my calorie deficit goal today."

Determine Your Optimal Macro-Nutrient Ratio
This kind of behavior will get you into trouble. You need to pay attention to how much processed food you are eating as opposed to natural foods and what proportion of your calories are coming from carbohydrates, protein and fat.

You should determine the best so called macro-nutrient ratio. For the average adult with a reasonably active lifestyle a ratio of 50-20-30 is recommended by most nutritionists. This means that about half of your calories should come from natural carbohydrates such as whole grains, vegetables, fruits, and beans.

Twenty percent of your calorie intake with this ratio would come from lean protein foods such as milk and wheat and cereal and thirty percent from dietary fat.

Regarding dietary fat you should watch the level of saturated vs. unsaturated fat and trans fat in your diet. Polyunsaturated and monounsaturated fats are good in your diet. Of course, the polyunsaturated fat you get from fish and nuts like walnuts are the best for your overall health because they help to reduce your cholesterol.

If you really want to drill down you can also keep track of nutrient values contained in the "energy calories" you eat in foods like protein, fat, alcohol and carbohydrates. You can also keep track of the amount of trans fat, salt, glucose, fiber and calcium. Then there are vitamins such as A, C, D, E, folic acid and selenium.

If you are this diligent in your counting you will know you are doing the best you can to fight diseases such a coronary heart disease, cancer, stroke and diabetes.

Pace Your Calorie Intake

It is way better to eat on a schedule so that your body is not hungry most of the time you are awake yet will still burn off the calories you eat daily and end the day with the calorie deficit you need in order to lose weight when you are ready to go to bed.

Probably the best schedule would be to try and eat an average size meal every four waking hours. Also, a technique that is often underemphasized is to minimize the calories you take in with beverages.

Rather than soft drinks and sodas you should drink water. In fact, you should drink enough water throughout the day so that your stomach feels full even when you are hungry. Plenty of water throughout the day will help your body to burn fat much more efficiently than without enough water.

Chapter 12

What You Have Learned So Far

Keep Score!

You probably are not losing weight because you are not keeping score or even paying attention to how many calories are going in and how many calories are getting burned off each day. You don't have a Smartphone app, handwritten log or online account to keep track of and count calories with. You have no idea how many calories you burn off every day with your routine of daily activities and exercise.

Well now you have some pretty good ideas of where to start no matter the level of your technical skill or desire to count your calories electronically with the latest technology.

Start By Knowing Your Maintenance Number

How many calories everyday does your body need to maintain your current weight? This number is critical to your weight loss program. End up the day with a net gain more than this number and you will be putting on weight not losing it. Achieving a caloric deficit every day will mean you are going to lose weight at a certain rate.

If you are not sure of what your maintenance calorie number is, a good way of finding out is to eat daily the number of calories you have determined as your maintenance level then weigh in first thing in the morning once per week to see if in fact you have remained at a stable weight. If you have gained weight then your maintenance estimate is too high. You will need to do this for two to three weeks at your normal level of physical activity.

Determining Your Daily Calorie Deficit

Now figure out how to keep ending the day with a deficit large enough to achieve your weight loss goal over the time period you have chosen. Repeat the process by cutting back on the amount of calorie intake by about 500 calories per day. At the end of this stage check to see if you have lost one or two pounds per week. It takes a calorie deficit of approximately 3500 calories to burn off one pound. So, add some good workout routines throughout the week and you may get to two pounds lost rather than one.

If you lose three pounds or more in one week you may be losing weight at a rate that is too fast. You want your weight loss program to be healthy and sustainable.

Your Customized Weight Loss Plan

Your goal should be achievable without starvation or excessive dangerous workouts taking into account your current health status. If your daily calorie deficit is too small then your weight loss will be so slow that you will not see any noticeable difference when you step on the scale and you will become discouraged.

On the other hand, if you are losing weight too fast you run the risk of not having enough energy to complete your exercise schedule and the risk of losing muscle in addition to fat. The commonly acceptable range in terms of pounds to lose each week for a sustainable and healthy weight loss program is from ½ to 2 pounds per week.

Your doctor, professional nutritionist, dietician and the other diet resources referred to above will help you come up with the best weight loss plan, optimal for your personal situation that will be sustainable over the long run and not subject your body and psyche to yo-yo diet fads.

If you Are Keeping Score You Can Adjust

It is a matter of small changes and incremental improvements. If you are not achieving your goals then you have to be willing to make adjustments. Perhaps different kinds of foods and different kinds of exercise will have to be added into your weight loss program.

Some people who count calories say "Eat whatever you want. As long as you are counting calories and you end up the day with your needed calorie deficit you are good to go". My opinion is that this will not work out in the long run and is not going to be healthy for you.

Obvious Food Adjustments You Can Make

If you are still eating things that are high in calories such as fast foods, sugary sodas, candy, cookies, ice cream, pastries, pies etc., then obviously there are adjustments you can make! When you log in the calorie count for these kinds of foods into whatever kind of calorie counter you have decided on, it should be obvious that these kinds of foods are "filling up" your daily calorie count.

Needless to say these kinds of foods in addition to making your weight loss goals much more difficult to achieve are also not healthy for you! Just eating a few chocolates, some Cheetos and a candy bar everyday is not going work! Go ahead and try it if you want to.

How Much To Adjust

So if you are not losing weight each week, a good strategy is to cut back on your daily calorie intake by approximately 250 to 300 calories per day each time you need to make an adjustment. Conversely, if you are losing too much weight, over three pounds per week, you should consider increasing your calorie intake by a similar amount.

Keep It Simple

Don't start out trying to make your weight loss program too complicated. I know we talked about the importance of eating healthy and keeping track of nutrients, carbs, sodium, trans fat, unsaturated and saturated fat, proteins, vitamins etc.; however, don't let this level of detailed tracking get you off track. Just start out with trying to achieve the best daily calorie deficit needed to achieve your weight loss goal. You can always get more detailed and more sophisticated in your tracking as you progress and your skills improve over time.

Also, don't get too fancy with your exercise routines and get confused with the best ratio of cardio vs. strength training, low vs. high impact etc. Just do what you can to start out and improve each day over time.

Being Held Accountable

How badly do you want to lose weight? How committed are you to getting on a program that will provide long term, steady and healthy weight loss that does not require a big cash outlay, periodic meetings and buying expensive name brand diet foods or unhealthy crash diets?

Where's The Pain?

So far I'll bet you are saying "I still don't see the PAIN you were talking about before! OK sure I've got a great diet plan and calorie counter taking advantage of the latest technology but it looks to me like I can STILL CHEAT pretty easily."

Yeah! That's why I am going to recommend that if at all possible, you go for the most tech savvy solution reviewed here and download the MyFitnessPal.com Calorie Counter and Diet Tracker App to your iPhone or Android Smartphone or use the UP wristband as a standalone calories counter. This way using the app you can check with your friends that are also using the app and monitor each other's progress. Don't worry if you have a phone run by windows or have a Blackberry, there are Calorie Counter apps for these also. This can also be done with the Jawbone UP wristband.

Who Are You Accountable To?

Being held accountable for your behavior is a crucial component in anything that requires self-discipline. By being part of a community that you can access anytime you need to and get the moral or even technical support you need, can make the difference between sticking with it and giving up. More importantly you know someone else will be monitoring your progress and will know if you are diet cheating. You will feel the pain of embarrassment "in front of the group" for cheating on your diet. If you don't feel the pain for cheating then what reason is there to share your progress with them?

If Using Your Smartphone Is Not Possible

Even if you have to "go it alone" without a Smartphone app you should still arrange for someone else to get involved with tracking your progress and having that person or group hold you accountable.

If you have the money and you need the extra help, hire a professional nutritionist or dietician as a consultant. This will not be inexpensive but you will get personal, individual and professional attention that could provide the motivation you need and result in the self-discipline you must have to avoid the diet cheater trap that is so discouraging for so many.

Chapter 13

It's Still Not Working!

Be Realistic
Some people start out with unrealistic expectations. Don't do this. Don't think you are going to lose twenty pounds in twenty days. Shoot for one to two pounds per week.

"Trying" Is Not Enough
If you are "trying" and it is not working then maybe you are not "doing" enough. By this I mean you have to DO what it takes to make your calorie counting program work. Get started – give it enough time to see if what you are doing is working (somewhere around three weeks) then make adjustments if it is not working. REPEAT!

The Latest Technology Will Make This Easier

Are you using technology to make calories counting as effortless as possible? If you are still using your Grandmother's system of weighing food, looking up calorie counts in books, adding up everything with a calculator and writing in a journal then you are NOT taking advantage of the latest technology and this might be slowing you down, discouraging you and causing you to fail. If you are actually successful doing it "the old fashion way" then great don't change what's working! But if you are not...time to gear up!

Too Much High Tech

"No, all this new technology is too confusing!" Well, that could certainly be the case if you are trying to count and track everything under the sun with multiple devices, several apps and two or more websites. Don't go down this route either. If you are a capable, savvy Smartphone user then find an app that suits your needs and can run on your Smartphone's operating system. Just make sure you can upload to the apps website and communicate with your support group.

On The Web Only

Standalone website calories counters can be good if you are not able to use your Smartphone for some reason or don't have one. This will be a little more time consuming and require more effort entering the data rather than scanning bar codes but the functionality will be as good as long as you choose a good site. Checkout the two we mentioned above. Going this way may make it more difficult to connect with your support group.

Can't Stop Cheating?

If you can't stop the cheating (you know what I mean don't say you don't) then your support system is not strong enough or you were not committed enough to begin with. Are you being held accountable by someone? Is that someone motivating you into the correct diet behavior? If you still really want this to work then make sure you are feeling enough "pain" when you fall off the course by eating that "one little cookie".

If embarrassment in front of your friends is not enough then condition your mind to "dread" some other punishment: Maybe doing some chore that you hate...over and over.   Or perhaps not getting rewarded with a pleasure you look forward to everyday.

You Have Reached A Plateau

If you have made your program work but now it is not working then you have to ask yourself, "What did I change?" Small changes in your daily routine can have a cumulative or compounding effect especially in your exercise and workout activity. Are you going out of town more than you were and don't have as much access to your exercise equipment? Have the last few months been filled up with an extra number of birthday cakes topped with ice cream?

Here is good question: If your previously working weight loss program was working but stopped, did you make big changes to the program unnecessarily? Some people just like change and want it whether it is warranted or not. Remember the old saying, "Don't argue with success". If you are achieving your goals then stick with what is working and don't let the latest and greatest technology or fad diet change your course.

Changing Muscle Groups

Some people get tripped up thinking they need to constantly "change up" their exercise routine or it will suddenly stop working. Well, change AFTER it stops working and not before.

Don't Skip Breakfast

Don't think that the best way to lower your calorie intake is to skip meals. This is especially true with your first meal of the day, breakfast. The old adage that breakfast is the most important meal of the day turns out to be right on. There are two very good reasons this is true. First of all, remember that your body has the entire day to burn off what you eat at breakfast. Remember, you are not usually going to go to bed and sleep a few hours after breakfast as you do with supper.

Also, you don't want to start out the day feeling hungry and remaining hungry until lunch or your first break before lunch. You will be tempted to eat more than you planned for at lunch or snack on something during your mid-morning break that you had not planned to eat at all. You want to start out the day as well as end the day "right" with your diet behavior.

Don't Skip Any Meals

This kind of "starvation logic" can even be carried out beyond breakfast when you decide to not only skip your first meal of the day but lunch also then eat hardly anything for supper. If you do this either because you are trying to lose weight too fast or because you are trying to "make up" for a "pig-out event" from yesterday, you will get hungrier and hungrier until you find yourself right in the middle of another pig-out.

Conclusion

Thanks for reading this book. I hope you were able to find some information that will be useful to you in your weight loss and calories counting effort. Please leave a review of this book. It would be greatly appreciated.

Then go over to:

http://www.weightlossextrabonus.com

and download your free weight loss bonus report. There is some great information in this report that there was just not enough room to cover here. You will also then be signed up to my newsletter that will update you on new information and resources related to calories counting and weight loss.

To download apps, discover other recommended weight loss reading, websites and browse other helpful resources visit:

http://www.weightlossextrabonus.com/resources

www.ingramcontent.com/pod-product-compliance
Lightning Source LLC
Chambersburg PA
CBHW070615290526
45790CB00002B/923